Organic Cooling Sprays
Top 40 Homemade Cool Down Spray Recipes To Beat The Heat

Table of content

Introduction

Today you find yourself under the shade of an old oak tree, soaking up the shade in your favorite hammock. You don't have a care in the world, and you don't have anything on your to do list. You have all the time to do anything and everything you want, but without any of the stress of a work day.

Yes, life is perfect, and you are left to enjoy yourself. Until it happens. Sure, it starts slow, but as it builds, you begin to feel more and more uncomfortable. You try moving to the left, then to the right. You try getting out of the hammock and embracing the coolness of the earth.

No matter what you try, you still have that uncomfortable feeling creeping up the back of your neck. You are hot. Looking up at the sunshine you can see why, for the sun is as bright and bold as it loves to be in the center of a summer day, but you are left to deal with the consequences, and they aren't pleasant.

So what do you do? You know you want to be outdoors, or you want to at least enjoy the open windows in your home while you can have them, but you don't like this sticky feeling that comes from the heat. There is only one thing to do, and that is to cool down.

But when you look at the sprays that are on the market today, you realize you are left with limited options. Whether you want something that is organic, or something that lacks any of the harmful chemicals you find in the other products on the market today, you know you have to figure out something, and soon.

That is the moment you reach for this book, and that is the moment everything changes for you. In this book, you are going to find everything you need to manage the heat, and beat the blaze. Get cool the fast and easy way when you use any one of these cooling sprays, and rest assured knowing they are all natural and organic, meaning you can use them without the stress.

So if you are ready to embrace the coolness while you are out in the summer sun, you have come to the right place. Get ready to cool down in a way you never thought possible before, and enjoy the summer for all that it has to offer.

Toss on your hat and head to the great outdoors.

Summer calls.

Chapter 1 – Just What the Doctor Ordered

The Ever Mist

15 drops peppermint oil

5 drops vanilla oil

5 drops lemon oil

1 cup distilled water

Directions:

Combine all ingredients in a small spray bottle.

You can either mix up a new batch of this cooling spray whenever you are in the mood to use it, or you can make and store in the fridge so it's always ready for you when you need it!

To use, simply spritz on your chest, arms, and legs. If you are going to use this on your forehead, I recommend you use it to dampen a wash cloth and gently apply from there.

You Had Me At Cool Down

15 drops hibiscus

5 drops chamomile

5 drops tea tree oil

1 cup distilled water

Directions:

Combine all ingredients in a small spray bottle.

You can either mix up a new batch of this cooling spray whenever you are in the mood to use it, or you can make and store in the fridge so it's always ready for you when you need it!

To use, simply spritz on your chest, arms, and legs. If you are going to use this on your forehead, I recommend you use it to dampen a wash cloth and gently apply from there.

A Chance Of Rain

20 drops jasmine oil

15 drops peppermint oil

5 drops wild orange oil

1 cup distilled water

Directions:

Combine all ingredients in a small spray bottle.

You can either mix up a new batch of this cooling spray whenever you are in the mood to use it, or you can make and store in the fridge so it's always ready for you when you need it!

To use, simply spritz on your chest, arms, and legs. If you are going to use this on your forehead, I recommend you use it to dampen a wash cloth and gently apply from there.

The Fantastic Four

5 drops fractionated coconut oil

5 drops jojoba oil

5 drops ylang ylang

5 drops lavender oil

1 cup distilled water

Directions:

Combine all ingredients in a small spray bottle.

You can either mix up a new batch of this cooling spray whenever you are in the mood to use it, or you can make and store in the fridge so it's always ready for you when you need it!

To use, simply spritz on your chest, arms, and legs. If you are going to use this on your forehead, I recommend you use it to dampen a wash cloth and gently apply from there.

Sunshine And Smiles

16 drops spearmint

4 drops peppermint oil

3 drops lavender oil

1 cup distilled water

Directions:

Combine all ingredients in a small spray bottle.

You can either mix up a new batch of this cooling spray whenever you are in the mood to use it, or you can make and store in the fridge so it's always ready for you when you need it!

To use, simply spritz on your chest, arms, and legs. If you are going to use this on your forehead, I recommend you use it to dampen a wash cloth and gently apply from there.

The Sun Blaster

10 drops Sunflower oil

5 drops rose oil

5 drops rose wood oil

1 cup distilled water

Directions:

Combine all ingredients in a small spray bottle.

You can either mix up a new batch of this cooling spray whenever you are in the mood to use it, or you can make and store in the fridge so it's always ready for you when you need it!

To use, simply spritz on your chest, arms, and legs. If you are going to use this on your forehead, I recommend you use it to dampen a wash cloth and gently apply from there.

A Lemon and a Lime

10 drops lemon oil

10 drops lemongrass oil

5 drops lime oil

1 cup distilled water

Directions:

Combine all ingredients in a small spray bottle.

You can either mix up a new batch of this cooling spray whenever you are in the mood to use it, or you can make and store in the fridge so it's always ready for you when you need it!

To use, simply spritz on your chest, arms, and legs. If you are going to use this on your forehead, I recommend you use it to dampen a wash cloth and gently apply from there.

A Day at the Parade

15 drops bubblegum aroma therapy oil

5 drops tea tree oil

5 drops peppermint oil

1 cup distilled water

Directions:

Combine all ingredients in a small spray bottle.

You can either mix up a new batch of this cooling spray whenever you are in the mood to use it, or you can make and store in the fridge so it's always ready for you when you need it!

To use, simply spritz on your chest, arms, and legs. If you are going to use this on your forehead, I recommend you use it to dampen a wash cloth and gently apply from there.

Chapter 2 – The Day Saver Recipes

The Spice Flower

10 drops hibiscus oil

10 drops ginger oil

5 drops basil

1 cup distilled water

Directions:

Combine all ingredients in a small spray bottle.

You can either mix up a new batch of this cooling spray whenever you are in the mood to use it, or you can make and store in the fridge so it's always ready for you when you need it!

To use, simply spritz on your chest, arms, and legs. If you are going to use this on your forehead, I recommend you use it to dampen a wash cloth and gently apply from there.

Call it What You Want

15 drops cinnamon oil

5 drops lavender

5 drops ginger oil

1 cup distilled water

Directions:

Combine all ingredients in a small spray bottle.

You can either mix up a new batch of this cooling spray whenever you are in the mood to use it, or you can make and store in the fridge so it's always ready for you when you need it!

To use, simply spritz on your chest, arms, and legs. If you are going to use this on your forehead, I recommend you use it to dampen a wash cloth and gently apply from there.

Hip Hip Hooray

18 drops rosewood oil

14 drops sandalwood oil

5 drops lilac oil

5 drops lavender oil

1 cup distilled water

Directions:

Combine all ingredients in a small spray bottle.

You can either mix up a new batch of this cooling spray whenever you are in the mood to use it, or you can make and store in the fridge so it's always ready for you when you need it!

To use, simply spritz on your chest, arms, and legs. If you are going to use this on your forehead, I recommend you use it to dampen a wash cloth and gently apply from there.

If You're Happy And You Know it

10 drops cotton candy aroma therapy oil

5 drops bubblegum aroma therapy oil

5 drops lemon oil

1 cup distilled water

Directions:

Combine all ingredients in a small spray bottle.

You can either mix up a new batch of this cooling spray whenever you are in the mood to use it, or you can make and store in the fridge so it's always ready for you when you need it!

To use, simply spritz on your chest, arms, and legs. If you are going to use this on your forehead, I recommend you use it to dampen a wash cloth and gently apply from there.

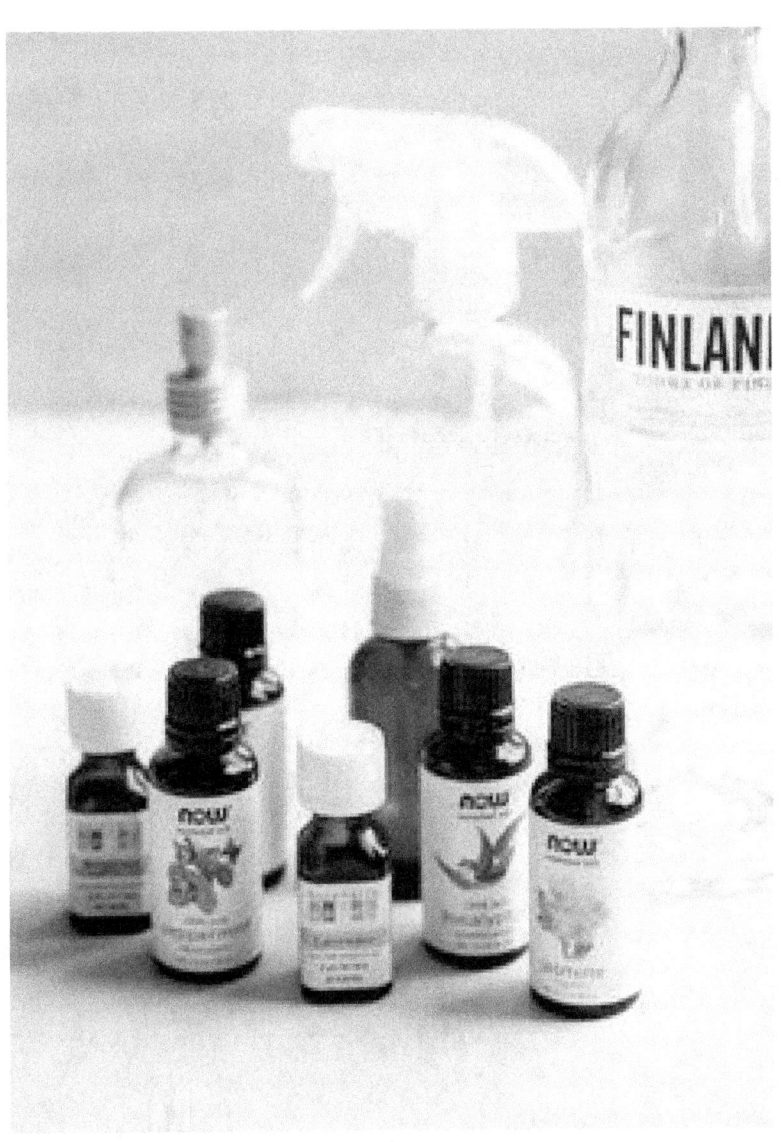

The Birthday Burst

10 drops bubblegum aroma therapy oil

10 drops cinnamon oil

10 drops peppermint oil

1 cup distilled water

Directions:

Combine all ingredients in a small spray bottle.

You can either mix up a new batch of this cooling spray whenever you are in the mood to use it, or you can make and store in the fridge so it's always ready for you when you need it!

To use, simply spritz on your chest, arms, and legs. If you are going to use this on your forehead, I recommend you use it to dampen a wash cloth and gently apply from there.

The Soothe Sayer

10 drops spearmint

10 drops mint

10 drops wintergreen

1 cup distilled water

Directions:

Combine all ingredients in a small spray bottle.

You can either mix up a new batch of this cooling spray whenever you are in the mood to use it, or you can make and store in the fridge so it's always ready for you when you need it!

To use, simply spritz on your chest, arms, and legs. If you are going to use this on your forehead, I recommend you use it to dampen a wash cloth and gently apply from there.

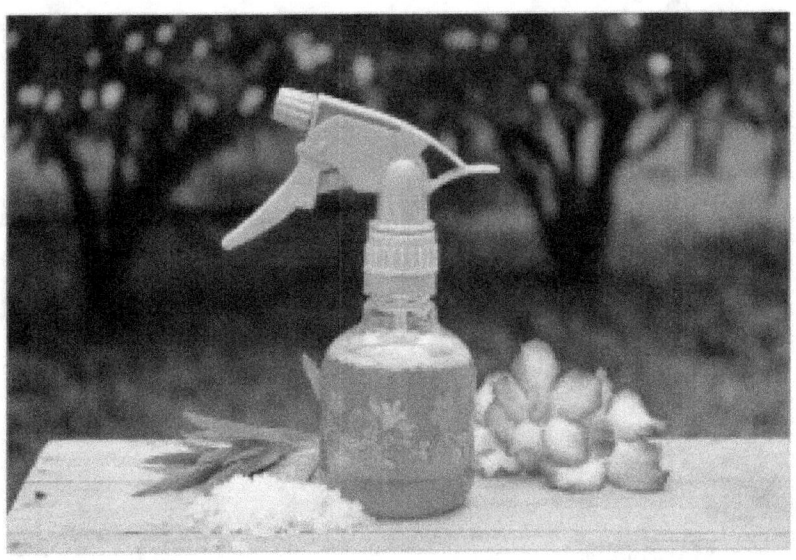

The Earthy Burst

10 drops patchouli oil

10 drops cedar

5 drops cedar wood

1 cup distilled water

Directions:

Combine all ingredients in a small spray bottle.

You can either mix up a new batch of this cooling spray whenever you are in the mood to use it, or you can make and store in the fridge so it's always ready for you when you need it!

To use, simply spritz on your chest, arms, and legs. If you are going to use this on your forehead, I recommend you use it to dampen a wash cloth and gently apply from there.

Wind in the Willows

10 drops wildflower aroma therapy oil

5 drops lemongrass

5 drops wheatgrass oil

1 cup distilled water

Directions:

Combine all ingredients in a small spray bottle.

You can either mix up a new batch of this cooling spray whenever you are in the mood to use it, or you can make and store in the fridge so it's always ready for you when you need it!

To use, simply spritz on your chest, arms, and legs. If you are going to use this on your forehead, I recommend you use it to dampen a wash cloth and gently apply from there.

Chapter 3 – Perfect Passion Mists

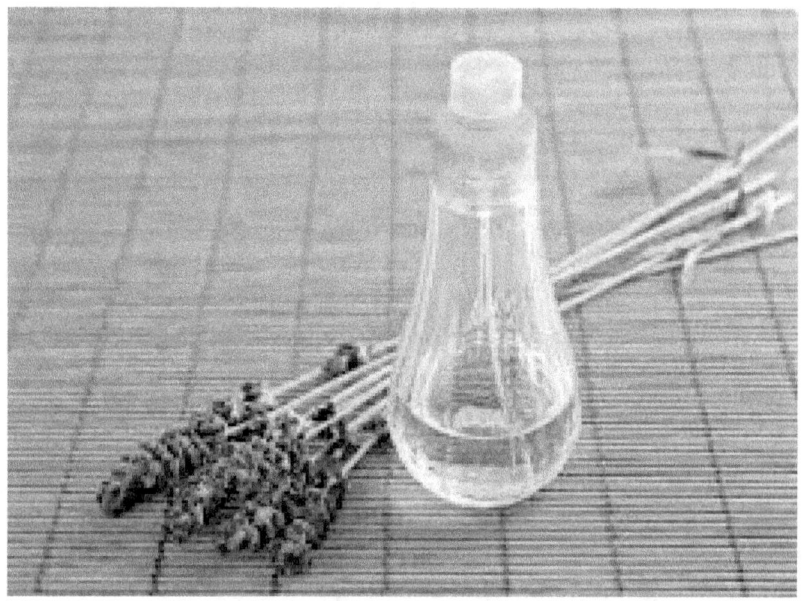

In the Name of Love

10 drops grapefruit

10 drops rose oil

10 drops orange oil

1 cup distilled water

Directions:

Combine all ingredients in a small spray bottle.

You can either mix up a new batch of this cooling spray whenever you are in the mood to use it, or you can make and store in the fridge so it's always ready for you when you need it!

To use, simply spritz on your chest, arms, and legs. If you are going to use this on your forehead, I recommend you use it to dampen a wash cloth and gently apply from there.

A Walk at the Park

10 drops dandelion oil

5 drops geranium oil

5 drops clove oil

5 drops pine oil

1 cup distilled water

Directions:

Combine all ingredients in a small spray bottle.

You can either mix up a new batch of this cooling spray whenever you are in the mood to use it, or you can make and store in the fridge so it's always ready for you when you need it!

To use, simply spritz on your chest, arms, and legs. If you are going to use this on your forehead, I recommend you use it to dampen a wash cloth and gently apply from there.

Frozen Citrus Burst

10 drops wintergreen

10 drops grapefruit

10 drops lemon

10 drops lime

5 drops blood orange

4 drops orange

1 cup distilled water

Directions:

Combine all ingredients in a small spray bottle.

You can either mix up a new batch of this cooling spray whenever you are in the mood to use it, or you can make and store in the fridge so it's always ready for you when you need it!

To use, simply spritz on your chest, arms, and legs. If you are going to use this on your forehead, I recommend you use it to dampen a wash cloth and gently apply from there.

The Morning Cooldown

10 drops frankincense

10 drops thieves oil

5 drops myrrh oil

1 cup distilled water

Directions:

Combine all ingredients in a small spray bottle.

You can either mix up a new batch of this cooling spray whenever you are in the mood to use it, or you can make and store in the fridge so it's always ready for you when you need it!

To use, simply spritz on your chest, arms, and legs. If you are going to use this on your forehead, I recommend you use it to dampen a wash cloth and gently apply from there.

The Prize Pack

10 drops Roman chamomile oil

10 drops ylang ylang

15 drops sandalwood

4 drops tea tree

1 cup distilled water

Directions:

Combine all ingredients in a small spray bottle.

You can either mix up a new batch of this cooling spray whenever you are in the mood to use it, or you can make and store in the fridge so it's always ready for you when you need it!

To use, simply spritz on your chest, arms, and legs. If you are going to use this on your forehead, I recommend you use it to dampen a wash cloth and gently apply from there.

To Be or Not to Be?

15 drops cardamom

10 drops ginger root oil

12 drops cedar

1 cup distilled water

Directions:

Combine all ingredients in a small spray bottle.

You can either mix up a new batch of this cooling spray whenever you are in the mood to use it, or you can make and store in the fridge so it's always ready for you when you need it!

To use, simply spritz on your chest, arms, and legs. If you are going to use this on your forehead, I recommend you use it to dampen a wash cloth and gently apply from there.

The Sexy Spritz

15 drops rose wood

10 drops grapefruit

10 drops white musk perfume oil

1 cup distilled water

Directions:

Combine all ingredients in a small spray bottle.

You can either mix up a new batch of this cooling spray whenever you are in the mood to use it, or you can make and store in the fridge so it's always ready for you when you need it!

To use, simply spritz on your chest, arms, and legs. If you are going to use this on your forehead, I recommend you use it to dampen a wash cloth and gently apply from there.

The Yes Man

10 drops wildflower aroma therapy oil

7 drops musk aroma therapy oil

8 drops pine

2 drops tea tree oil

1 cup distilled water

Directions:

Combine all ingredients in a small spray bottle.

You can either mix up a new batch of this cooling spray whenever you are in the mood to use it, or you can make and store in the fridge so it's always ready for you when you need it!

To use, simply spritz on your chest, arms, and legs. If you are going to use this on your forehead, I recommend you use it to dampen a wash cloth and gently apply from there.

Chapter 4 – The Heater Beaters

Cool Misty Forest

10 drops cedar

10 drops pine

10 drops spearmint

1 cup distilled water

Directions:

Combine all ingredients in a small spray bottle.

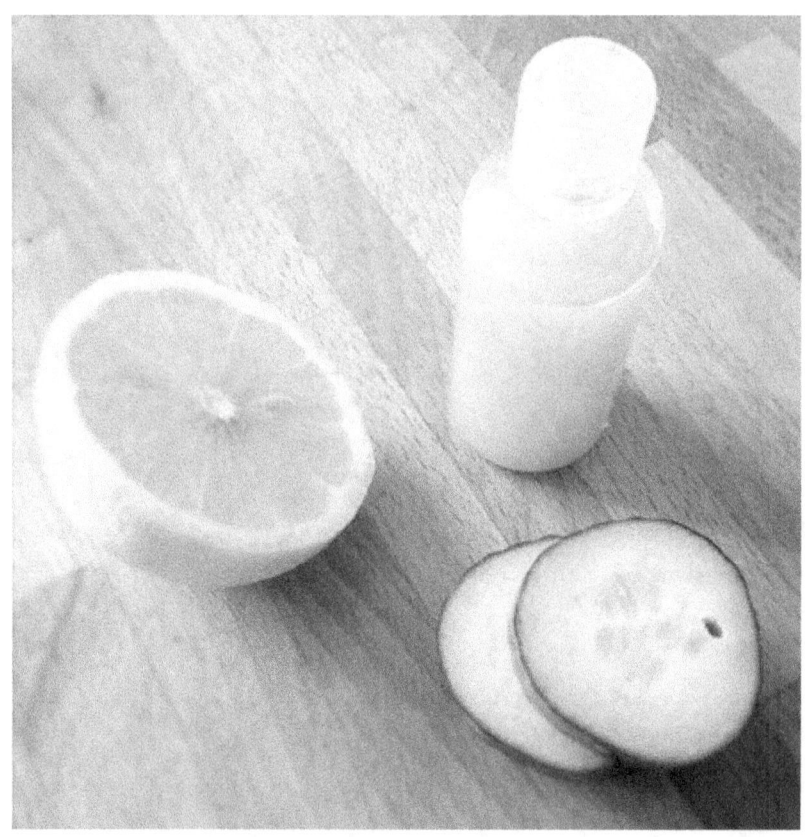

You can either mix up a new batch of this cooling spray whenever you are in the mood to use it, or you can make and store in the fridge so it's always ready for you when you need it!

To use, simply spritz on your chest, arms, and legs. If you are going to use this on your forehead, I recommend you use it to dampen a wash cloth and gently apply from there.

Winter Rush

10 drops peppermint

10 drops wintergreen

10 drops mint

10 drops eucalyptus

1 cup distilled water

Directions:

Combine all ingredients in a small spray bottle.

You can either mix up a new batch of this cooling spray whenever you are in the mood to use it, or you can make and store in the fridge so it's always ready for you when you need it!

To use, simply spritz on your chest, arms, and legs. If you are going to use this on your forehead, I recommend you use it to dampen a wash cloth and gently apply from there.

Catching Waves

10 drops eucalyptus

8 drops chamomile

10 drops bergamot

1 cup distilled water

Directions:

Combine all ingredients in a small spray bottle.

You can either mix up a new batch of this cooling spray whenever you are in the mood to use it, or you can make and store in the fridge so it's always ready for you when you need it!

To use, simply spritz on your chest, arms, and legs. If you are going to use this on your forehead, I recommend you use it to dampen a wash cloth and gently apply from there.

Also a great soothing mist to use on sunburns, simply hold the spray bottle a few inches away from the burn, and gently mist.

Any time you need that cool burst of refreshment, just spritz away!

The Bare Necessities

10 drops myrrh

10 drops rose wood

5 drops patchouli

5 drops ylang ylang

1 cup distilled water

Directions:

Combine all ingredients in a small spray bottle.

You can either mix up a new batch of this cooling spray whenever you are in the mood to use it, or you can make and store in the fridge so it's always ready for you when you need it!

To use, simply spritz on your chest, arms, and legs. If you are going to use this on your forehead, I recommend you use it to dampen a wash cloth and gently apply from there.

Three's a Crowd

10 drops green meadow aroma therapy oil

10 drops myrrh

10 drops goldenseal oil

1 cup distilled water

Directions:

Combine all ingredients in a small spray bottle.

You can either mix up a new batch of this cooling spray whenever you are in the mood to use it, or you can make and store in the fridge so it's always ready for you when you need it!

To use, simply spritz on your chest, arms, and legs. If you are going to use this on your forehead, I recommend you use it to dampen a wash cloth and gently apply from there.

A Day At Carnival Avenue

10 drops popcorn aroma therapy oil

5 drops cotton candy aroma therapy oil

5 drops thieves oil

1 cup distilled water

Directions:

Combine all ingredients in a small spray bottle.

You can either mix up a new batch of this cooling spray whenever you are in the mood to use it, or you can make and store in the fridge so it's always ready for you when you need it!

To use, simply spritz on your chest, arms, and legs. If you are going to use this on your forehead, I recommend you use it to dampen a wash cloth and gently apply from there.

Running Through The Streets

10 drops cedarwood

10 drops rose wood

10 drops wood blend essential oil

5 drops patchouli

1 cup distilled water

Directions:

Combine all ingredients in a small spray bottle.

You can either mix up a new batch of this cooling spray whenever you are in the mood to use it, or you can make and store in the fridge so it's always ready for you when you need it!

To use, simply spritz on your chest, arms, and legs. If you are going to use this on your forehead, I recommend you use it to dampen a wash cloth and gently apply from there.

To Freedom

10 drops linen aroma therapy oil

10 drops lilac essential oil

5 drops lavender oil

1 cup distilled water

Directions:

Combine all ingredients in a small spray bottle.

You can either mix up a new batch of this cooling spray whenever you are in the mood to use it, or you can make and store in the fridge so it's always ready for you when you need it!

To use, simply spritz on your chest, arms, and legs. If you are going to use this on your forehead, I recommend you use it to dampen a wash cloth and gently apply from there.

Chapter 5 – The Best of the Rest

The One and Only

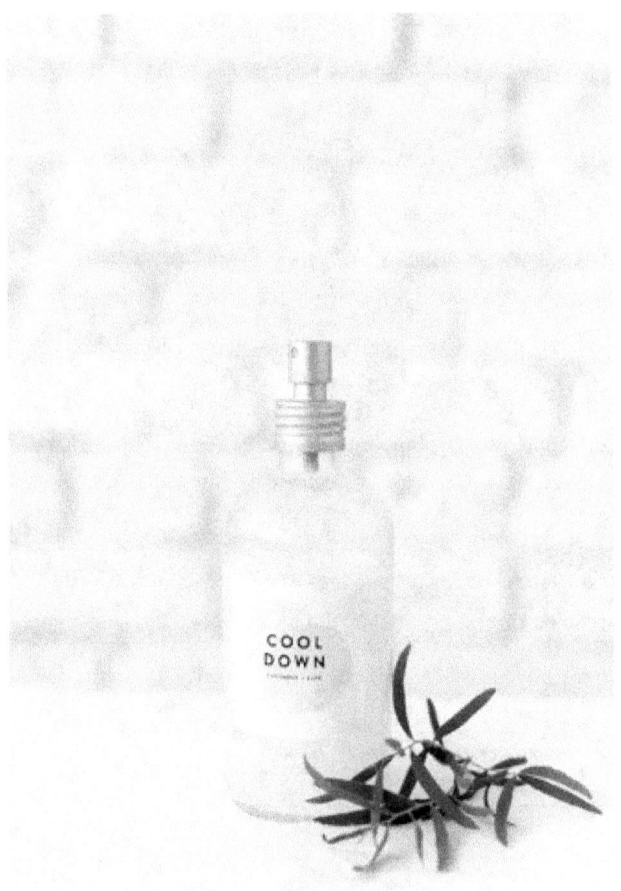

15 drops eucalyptus

10 drops grapefruit

10 drops mint

1 cup distilled water

Directions:

Combine all ingredients in a small spray bottle.

You can either mix up a new batch of this cooling spray whenever you are in the mood to use it, or you can make and store in the fridge so it's always ready for you when you need it!

To use, simply spritz on your chest, arms, and legs. If you are going to use this on your forehead, I recommend you use it to dampen a wash cloth and gently apply from there.

Brining Style Back

10 drops basil oi

10 drops ginger oil

10 drops coriander oil

1 cup distilled water

Directions:

Combine all ingredients in a small spray bottle.

You can either mix up a new batch of this cooling spray whenever you are in the mood to use it, or you can make and store in the fridge so it's always ready for you when you need it!

To use, simply spritz on your chest, arms, and legs. If you are going to use this on your forehead, I recommend you use it to dampen a wash cloth and gently apply from there.

You Plus Me

10 drops thieves oil

10 drops frankincense oil

5 drops tea tree oil

5 drops German Chamomile

1 cup distilled water

Directions:

Combine all ingredients in a small spray bottle.

You can either mix up a new batch of this cooling spray whenever you are in the mood to use it, or you can make and store in the fridge so it's always ready for you when you need it!

To use, simply spritz on your chest, arms, and legs. If you are going to use this on your forehead, I recommend you use it to dampen a wash cloth and gently apply from there.

The Cool Cat

10 drops geranium oil

10 drops lavender

10 drops hibiscus oil

10 drops grapefruit oil

1 cup distilled water

Directions:

Combine all ingredients in a small spray bottle.

You can either mix up a new batch of this cooling spray whenever you are in the mood to use it, or you can make and store in the fridge so it's always ready for you when you need it!

To use, simply spritz on your chest, arms, and legs. If you are going to use this on your forehead, I recommend you use it to dampen a wash cloth and gently apply from there.

Icy Blast

10 drops spearmint

10 drops pine

10 drops lemon oil

10 drops lime

1 cup distilled water

Directions:

Combine all ingredients in a small spray bottle.

You can either mix up a new batch of this cooling spray whenever you are in the mood to use it, or you can make and store in the fridge so it's always ready for you when you need it!

To use, simply spritz on your chest, arms, and legs. If you are going to use this on your forehead, I recommend you use it to dampen a wash cloth and gently apply from there.

Do That Up

10 drops ylang ylang

10 drops vanilla

10 drops white musk perfume oil

1 cup distilled water

Directions:

Combine all ingredients in a small spray bottle.

You can either mix up a new batch of this cooling spray whenever you are in the mood to use it, or you can make and store in the fridge so it's always ready for you when you need it!

To use, simply spritz on your chest, arms, and legs. If you are going to use this on your forehead, I recommend you use it to dampen a wash cloth and gently apply from there.

The Cure All

10 drops peppermint

10 drops rose

10 drops patchouli

10 drops frankincense

5 drops myrrh

1 cup distilled water

Directions:

Combine all ingredients in a small spray bottle.

You can either mix up a new batch of this cooling spray whenever you are in the mood to use it, or you can make and store in the fridge so it's always ready for you when you need it!

To use, simply spritz on your chest, arms, and legs. If you are going to use this on your forehead, I recommend you use it to dampen a wash cloth and gently apply from there.

Around the World in Eight Minutes

10 drops ginger root

4 drops thieves oil

4 drops tea tree oil

4 drops carrot seed oil

4 drops blood orange oil

1 cup distilled water

Directions:

Combine all ingredients in a small spray bottle.

You can either mix up a new batch of this cooling spray whenever you are in the mood to use it, or you can make and store in the fridge so it's always ready for you when you need it!

To use, simply spritz on your chest, arms, and legs. If you are going to use this on your forehead, I recommend you use it to dampen a wash cloth and gently apply from there.

Conclusion

There you have it, everything you need to beat the heat in style. Whether you want something subtle and sweet, or if you are ready to grab something that is wild and fresh, you are going to find what you need in the recipes in this book.

I hope this book was able to show you how you can beat the heat the easy way, and forget about the stress of spraying your body with all kinds of chemicals that you don't want anywhere near your skin.

This book is designed to help you enjoy your summer and feel good as you do it. Don't worry about how hot the thermometer reads, and don't worry about how you are going to handle the heat waves that are destined to be on their way the first of the week.

When you have a handy spray within your arm's reach, you have everything you need to take your summer fun to the next level. There's nothing stopping you from putting yourself out there and diving into all summer has to offer, and the more you are able to protect yourself from the exhausting heat, the better off you are going to be all around.

So are you ready to grab a bottle of cooling spray? Are you ready to arm yourself with everything you need to make your summer as enjoyable as you wanted it to be? If you are ready to ditch the sticky disaster of dealing with this heat on your own, then whip up any one of these recipes today, and you are going to have everything you need to enjoy summer as it was meant to be enjoyed.

What are you waiting for? Summer is going to end before you know it, and you don't want to be left sunburned in the heat. Grab your bottles and mix up your recipes... this is going to be the best summer you can imagine.

FREE Bonus Reminder

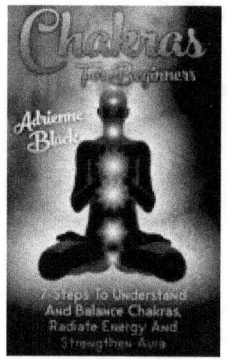

If you have not grabbed it yet, please go ahead and download your special bonus E book *"Chakras for Beginners. 7 Steps To Understand And Balance Chakras, Radiate Energy, And Strengthen Aura"*.

Simply Click the Button Below

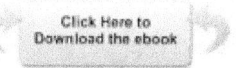

OR Go to This Page

http://lifehacksworld.com/free

BONUS #2: More Free & Discounted Books & Products

Do you want to receive more Free/Discounted Books or Products?

We have a mailing list where we send out our new Books or Products when they go free or with a discount on Amazon. Click on the link below to sign up for Free & Discount Book & Product Promotions.

=> **Sign Up for Free & Discount Book & Product Promotions** <=

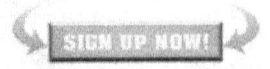

OR Go to this URL

http://zbit.ly/1WBb1Ek